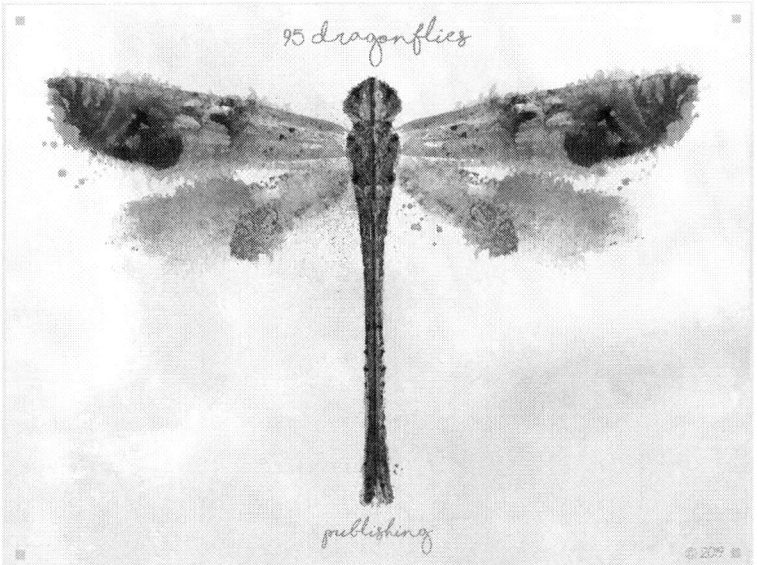

95 dragonflies

publishing

First edition, August, 2019

ISBN: 978-0-578-59135-3

"I don't want to be at the mercy of my emotions. I want to use them, to enjoy them, and to dominate them." - *Oscar Wilde*

Welcome to the

Who's Driving Your Bus Emotions Journal!

My intention for this journal is to provide you with a place to explore, track and learn about your emotions. We are all very similar yet our interpretation of the world around us and the nuance within those interpretations make us very different. Without an understanding of our many bus drivers, we will continue to be hijacked and driven around haphazardly.

Eleanor Roosevelt said *"No one can make you feel inferior without your consent."* This quote is spot on. When we unconsciously allow others onto our bus, we are giving up our power, the power to choose the emotions that serve us best.

As the saying goes, when you know better, you can do better.

Awareness is the fuel for change. Questions heighten your awareness. BE CURIOUS.

Let's fuel your bus up and get going!

As a reminder from Who's Driving Your Bus?,

the 'In-The-Moment Strategy' looks like this: You feel your emotions going up. You immediately:

To simplify the process, the 'In-The-Moment Strategy' looks like this:

You feel your emotions going up. You immediately...

!. STOP - Actually tell yourself to stop.

2. REFLECT - Breathe. get back into the current moment. Heighten your awareness - "Who is the current driver?"

3. CHOOSE - Ask yourself "Who is a better driver right now ?" Be mindful of your desired outcome.

4. REDIRECT - Once you have awareness, choose a different driver if need be.

REMEMBER, the secret sauce is made up of awareness, choice, action, and consistency.

THE 72 Hour Challenge

Whether you have just finished reading the book or you have just jumped to this section before you started the book, the 72 Hour Challenge is a major component to achieving success in managing your emotions.

Becoming aware of what is going on in your head, how your emotions are affecting you and how often this happens is the foundation to change.

If you would like to watch the video, please go to authorkimjohnson.com/72hourchallenge for an in-depth explanation.

If you would like to dive in, the steps are as follows:

1. Ask yourself if you are honestly committed to the ENTIRE 72 hours of the challenge. It takes the commitment of being "all in" in order not to quit when it gets tough and you become frustrated.

2. Decide how you will record your tracking. I am a big fan of thought capturing in a small note book. However a notes app or texting yourself are also strategies that my clients utilize.

3. Before the 72 hours begin, sit down and write out all the emotions you believe you experience during the day. Really think about your day, your week and remember how your emotions transitioned.

4. Write out any situations and/or people that push your buttons and that trigger your emotions.

5. Set your 72 hour start time. It's best to begin when you get out bed. Immediately notice which emotion you are experiencing while waking up.

6. From the moment you wake up till the moment you go to sleep, every time that you are aware of the emotion you are in, record it. Be aware that emotions change rapidly and often. This is the very reason that this exercise require patience with yourself. While it is a simple exercise, it is certainly not easy!

7. You will most likely notice that you stay within a small selection of emotions, looping through 3 - 5 different ones. This is very normal.

8. As you become aware of your emotions, you will begin to find them shifting by the very act of identifying them.

9. During this challenge, stay consistent with identifying as many as you can. The point is to find out how much time you stay in particular emotions and how much that emotion restricts your progress.

10. Ask yourself if the emotion you are experiencing is serving you. By recognizing whether or not the emotion is serving you, you can begin to see the reason this exercise is so helpful.

11. Laugh at yourself. Find humor in the way your mind and emotions are working. It's inevitable that you will judge yourself for how you feel. Again, that's perfectly fine. It's all very normal.

12. Keep up the recording for the entire 72 hours so you have a solid record of where your emotions go. Give yourself the gift of knowing what goes on in your head.

If you have already read the book, you can layer the 72 hours like Lily in the story, identify and shifting your emotions. Whether you decide to just identify your emotions in the first 72 hours or identify and shift your emotions as Lily did, you will come to a new level of awareness.

Remember, this should be fun! Don't be so hard on yourself and again, be patient. You've got this!

Have you started thinking about who your primary driver(s) is/are?

_____

_____

_____

_____

_____

_____

_____

_____

_____

_____

_____

_____

_____

_____

_____

_____

Who are the different emotions that drive your bus during a day?

_____

_____

_____

_____

_____

_____

_____

_____

_____

_____

_____

_____

_____

_____

_____

_____

_____

What will you name your drivers?

What can you learn about your drivers? What triggers them to show up?

_____

_____

_____

_____

_____

_____

_____

_____

_____

_____

_____

_____

_____

_____

_____

_____

Who are your top 3 - 5 primary drivers?

Who will your favorite CHOSEN driver be?

_____

_____

_____

_____

_____

_____

_____

_____

_____

_____

_____

_____

_____

_____

_____

_____

_____

_____

_____

_____

"You've always had the power my dear, you just had to learn it for yourself." - *Glinda, The Wizard Of Oz*

Date ....

What emotion/s were driving when you woke up today?

....

....

What emotion/s did I choose to be my driver for my
morning?

....

....

Did my emotions get triggered today and hijack my
bus? If so, what was the trigger?

....

....

What drivers did I chose throughout my day? Were
they my most resourceful drivers?

....

....

What emotion did I chose as my driver when I came
home today?

....

....

What emotion did I choose to end my day?

....

....

Date ....

Random thoughts about your bus today:

....

....

....

....

....

....

....

....

....

....

....

....

....

....

....

....

....

....

....

Date ....

What emotion/s were driving when you woke up today?

....

....

What emotion/s did I choose to be my driver for my
morning?

....

....

Did my emotions get triggered today and hijack my
bus? If so, what was the trigger?

....

....

What drivers did I chose throughout my day? Were
they my most resourceful drivers?

....

....

What emotion did I chose as my driver when I came
home today?

....

....

What emotion did I choose to end my day?

....

....

Date ....

Random thoughts about your bus today:

....

....

....

....

....

....

....

....

....

....

....

....

....

....

....

....

....

....

....

Date ....

What emotion/s were driving when you woke up today?

....

....

What emotion/s did I choose to be my driver for my morning?

....

....

Did my emotions get triggered today and hijack my bus? If so, what was the trigger?

....

....

What drivers did I chose throughout my day? Were they my most resourceful drivers?

....

....

What emotion did I chose as my driver when I came home today?

....

....

What emotion did I choose to end my day?

....

....

Date ....

Random thoughts about your bus today:

....

....

....

....

....

....

....

....

....

....

....

....

....

....

....

....

....

....

....

....

Date ....

What emotion/s were driving when you woke up today?

....

....

What emotion/s did I choose to be my driver for my morning?

....

....

Did my emotions get triggered today and hijack my bus? If so, what was the trigger?

....

....

What drivers did I chose throughout my day? Were they my most resourceful drivers?

....

....

What emotion did I chose as my driver when I came home today?

....

....

What emotion did I choose to end my day?

....

....

Date ....

Random thoughts about your bus today:

....

....

....

....

....

....

....

....

....

....

....

....

....

....

....

....

....

....

....

....

Date ....

What emotion/s were driving when you woke up today?

....

....

What emotion/s did I choose to be my driver for my morning?

....

....

Did my emotions get triggered today and hijack my bus? If so, what was the trigger?

....

....

What drivers did I chose throughout my day? Were they my most resourceful drivers?

....

....

What emotion did I chose as my driver when I came home today?

....

....

What emotion did I choose to end my day?

....

....

Date ....

Random thoughts about your bus today:

....

....

....

....

....

....

....

....

....

....

....

....

....

....

....

....

....

....

....

Date ....

What emotion/s were driving when you woke up today?

....

....

What emotion/s did I choose to be my driver for my morning?

....

....

Did my emotions get triggered today and hijack my bus? If so, what was the trigger?

....

....

What drivers did I chose throughout my day? Were they my most resourceful drivers?

....

....

What emotion did I chose as my driver when I came home today?

....

....

What emotion did I choose to end my day?

....

....

Date ....

Random thoughts about your bus today:

....
....
....
....
....
....
....
....
....
....
....
....
....
....
....
....
....
....
....
....

Date ....

What emotion/s were driving when you woke up today?

....

....

What emotion/s did I choose to be my driver for my morning?

....

....

Did my emotions get triggered today and hijack my bus? If so, what was the trigger?

....

....

What drivers did I chose throughout my day? Were they my most resourceful drivers?

....

....

What emotion did I chose as my driver when I came home today?

....

....

What emotion did I choose to end my day?

....

....

Date ....

Random thoughts about your bus today:

....

....

....

....

....

....

....

....

....

....

....

....

....

....

....

....

....

....

....

....

Date ....

What emotion/s were driving when you woke up today?

....

....

What emotion/s did I choose to be my driver for my morning?

....

....

Did my emotions get triggered today and hijack my bus? If so, what was the trigger?

....

....

What drivers did I chose throughout my day? Were they my most resourceful drivers?

....

....

What emotion did I chose as my driver when I came home today?

....

....

What emotion did I choose to end my day?

....

....

Date ....

Random thoughts about your bus today:

....

....

....

....

....

....

....

....

....

....

....

....

....

....

....

....

....

....

....

....

Date ....

What emotion/s were driving when you woke up today?

....

....

What emotion/s did I choose to be my driver for my morning?

....

....

Did my emotions get triggered today and hijack my bus? If so, what was the trigger?

....

....

What drivers did I chose throughout my day? Were they my most resourceful drivers?

....

....

What emotion did I chose as my driver when I came home today?

....

....

What emotion did I choose to end my day?

....

....

Date ....

Random thoughts about your bus today:

....

....

....

....

....

....

....

....

....

....

....

....

....

....

....

....

....

....

....

....

Date ....

What emotion/s were driving when you woke up today?

....

....

What emotion/s did I choose to be my driver for my morning?

....

....

Did my emotions get triggered today and hijack my bus? If so, what was the trigger?

....

....

What drivers did I chose throughout my day? Were they my most resourceful drivers?

....

....

What emotion did I chose as my driver when I came home today?

....

....

What emotion did I choose to end my day?

....

....

Date ....

Random thoughts about your bus today:

....

....

....

....

....

....

....

....

....

....

....

....

....

....

....

....

....

....

....

Date ....

What emotion/s were driving when you woke up today?

....

....

What emotion/s did I choose to be my driver for my morning?

....

....

Did my emotions get triggered today and hijack my bus? If so, what was the trigger?

....

....

What drivers did I chose throughout my day? Were they my most resourceful drivers?

....

....

What emotion did I chose as my driver when I came home today?

....

....

What emotion did I choose to end my day?

....

....

Date ....

Random thoughts about your bus today:

....

....

....

....

....

....

....

....

....

....

....

....

....

....

....

....

....

....

....

....

Date ....

What emotion/s were driving when you woke up today?

....

....

What emotion/s did I choose to be my driver for my morning?

....

....

Did my emotions get triggered today and hijack my bus? If so, what was the trigger?

....

....

What drivers did I chose throughout my day? Were they my most resourceful drivers?

....

....

What emotion did I chose as my driver when I came home today?

....

....

What emotion did I choose to end my day?

....

....

Date ....

Random thoughts about your bus today:

....

....

....

....

....

....

....

....

....

....

....

....

....

....

....

....

....

....

....

....

Date ....

What emotion/s were driving when you woke up today?

....

....

What emotion/s did I choose to be my driver for my morning?

....

....

Did my emotions get triggered today and hijack my bus? If so, what was the trigger?

....

....

What drivers did I chose throughout my day? Were they my most resourceful drivers?

....

....

What emotion did I chose as my driver when I came home today?

....

....

What emotion did I choose to end my day?

....

....

Date ....

Random thoughts about your bus today:

....

....

....

....

....

....

....

....

....

....

....

....

....

....

....

....

....

....

....

Date ....

What emotion/s were driving when you woke up today?

....

....

What emotion/s did I choose to be my driver for my morning?

....

....

Did my emotions get triggered today and hijack my bus? If so, what was the trigger?

....

....

What drivers did I chose throughout my day? Were they my most resourceful drivers?

....

....

What emotion did I chose as my driver when I came home today?

....

....

What emotion did I choose to end my day?

....

....

Date ....

Random thoughts about your bus today:

....

....

....

....

....

....

....

....

....

....

....

....

....

....

....

....

....

....

....

....

Date ....

What emotion/s were driving when you woke up today?

....

....

What emotion/s did I choose to be my driver for my
morning?

....

....

Did my emotions get triggered today and hijack my
bus? If so, what was the trigger?

....

....

What drivers did I chose throughout my day? Were
they my most resourceful drivers?

....

....

What emotion did I chose as my driver when I came
home today?

....

....

What emotion did I choose to end my day?

....

....

Date ....

Random thoughts about your bus today:

....

....

....

....

....

....

....

....

....

....

....

....

....

....

....

....

....

....

....

....

Date ....

What emotion/s were driving when you woke up today?

....

....

What emotion/s did I choose to be my driver for my
morning?

....

....

Did my emotions get triggered today and hijack my
bus? If so, what was the trigger?

....

....

What drivers did I chose throughout my day? Were
they my most resourceful drivers?

....

....

What emotion did I chose as my driver when I came
home today?

....

....

What emotion did I choose to end my day?

....

....

Date ....

Random thoughts about your bus today:

....

....

....

....

....

....

....

....

....

....

....

....

....

....

....

....

....

....

....

....

Date ....

What emotion/s were driving when you woke up today?

....

....

What emotion/s did I choose to be my driver for my morning?

....

....

Did my emotions get triggered today and hijack my bus? If so, what was the trigger?

....

....

What drivers did I chose throughout my day? Were they my most resourceful drivers?

....

....

What emotion did I chose as my driver when I came home today?

....

....

What emotion did I choose to end my day?

....

....

Date ....

Random thoughts about your bus today:

....

....

....

....

....

....

....

....

....

....

....

....

....

....

....

....

....

....

....

Date ....

What emotion/s were driving when you woke up today?

....

....

What emotion/s did I choose to be my driver for my
morning?

....

....

Did my emotions get triggered today and hijack my
bus? If so, what was the trigger?

....

....

What drivers did I chose throughout my day? Were
they my most resourceful drivers?

....

....

What emotion did I chose as my driver when I came
home today?

....

....

What emotion did I choose to end my day?

....

....

Date ....

Random thoughts about your bus today:

....

....

....

....

....

....

....

....

....

....

....

....

....

....

....

....

....

....

....

Date ....

What emotion/s were driving when you woke up today?

....

....

What emotion/s did I choose to be my driver for my morning?

....

....

Did my emotions get triggered today and hijack my bus? If so, what was the trigger?

....

....

What drivers did I chose throughout my day? Were they my most resourceful drivers?

....

....

What emotion did I chose as my driver when I came home today?

....

....

What emotion did I choose to end my day?

....

....

Date ....

Random thoughts about your bus today:

....

....

....

....

....

....

....

....

....

....

....

....

....

....

....

....

....

....

....

Date ....

What emotion/s were driving when you woke up today?

....

....

What emotion/s did I choose to be my driver for my morning?

....

....

Did my emotions get triggered today and hijack my bus? If so, what was the trigger?

....

....

What drivers did I chose throughout my day? Were they my most resourceful drivers?

....

....

What emotion did I chose as my driver when I came home today?

....

....

What emotion did I choose to end my day?

....

....

Date ....

Random thoughts about your bus today:

....

....

....

....

....

....

....

....

....

....

....

....

....

....

....

....

....

....

....

....

Date ....

What emotion/s were driving when you woke up today?

....

....

What emotion/s did I choose to be my driver for my
morning?

....

....

Did my emotions get triggered today and hijack my
bus? If so, what was the trigger?

....

....

What drivers did I chose throughout my day? Were
they my most resourceful drivers?

....

....

What emotion did I chose as my driver when I came
home today?

....

....

What emotion did I choose to end my day?

....

....

Date ....

Random thoughts about your bus today:

....

....

....

....

....

....

....

....

....

....

....

....

....

....

....

....

....

....

....

....

Date ....

What emotion/s were driving when you woke up today?

....

....

What emotion/s did I choose to be my driver for my morning?

....

....

Did my emotions get triggered today and hijack my bus? If so, what was the trigger?

....

....

What drivers did I chose throughout my day? Were they my most resourceful drivers?

....

....

What emotion did I chose as my driver when I came home today?

....

....

What emotion did I choose to end my day?

....

....

Date ....

Random thoughts about your bus today:

....
....
....
....
....
....
....
....
....
....
....
....
....
....
....
....
....
....
....
....

Date ....

What emotion/s were driving when you woke up today?

....

....

What emotion/s did I choose to be my driver for my morning?

....

....

Did my emotions get triggered today and hijack my bus? If so, what was the trigger?

....

....

What drivers did I chose throughout my day? Were they my most resourceful drivers?

....

....

What emotion did I chose as my driver when I came home today?

....

....

What emotion did I choose to end my day?

....

....

Date ....

Random thoughts about your bus today:

....

....

....

....

....

....

....

....

....

....

....

....

....

....

....

....

....

....

....

....

Date ....

What emotion/s were driving when you woke up today?

....

....

What emotion/s did I choose to be my driver for my morning?

....

....

Did my emotions get triggered today and hijack my bus? If so, what was the trigger?

....

....

What drivers did I chose throughout my day? Were they my most resourceful drivers?

....

....

What emotion did I chose as my driver when I came home today?

....

....

What emotion did I choose to end my day?

....

....

Date ....

Random thoughts about your bus today:

....

....

....

....

....

....

....

....

....

....

....

....

....

....

....

....

....

....

....

....

Date ....

What emotion/s were driving when you woke up today?

....

....

What emotion/s did I choose to be my driver for my morning?

....

....

Did my emotions get triggered today and hijack my bus? If so, what was the trigger?

....

....

What drivers did I chose throughout my day? Were they my most resourceful drivers?

....

....

What emotion did I chose as my driver when I came home today?

....

....

What emotion did I choose to end my day?

....

....

Date ....

Random thoughts about your bus today:

....

....

....

....

....

....

....

....

....

....

....

....

....

....

....

....

....

....

....

....

Date ....

What emotion/s were driving when you woke up today?

....

....

What emotion/s did I choose to be my driver for my
morning?

....

....

Did my emotions get triggered today and hijack my
bus? If so, what was the trigger?

....

....

What drivers did I chose throughout my day? Were
they my most resourceful drivers?

....

....

What emotion did I chose as my driver when I came
home today?

....

....

What emotion did I choose to end my day?

....

....

Date ....

Random thoughts about your bus today:

....

....

....

....

....

....

....

....

....

....

....

....

....

....

....

....

....

....

....

Date ....

What emotion/s were driving when you woke up today?

....

....

What emotion/s did I choose to be my driver for my morning?

....

....

Did my emotions get triggered today and hijack my bus? If so, what was the trigger?

....

....

What drivers did I chose throughout my day? Were they my most resourceful drivers?

....

....

What emotion did I chose as my driver when I came home today?

....

....

What emotion did I choose to end my day?

....

....

Date ....

Random thoughts about your bus today:

....

....

....

....

....

....

....

....

....

....

....

....

....

....

....

....

....

....

....

....

Date ....

What emotion/s were driving when you woke up today?

....

....

What emotion/s did I choose to be my driver for my morning?

....

....

Did my emotions get triggered today and hijack my bus? If so, what was the trigger?

....

....

What drivers did I chose throughout my day? Were they my most resourceful drivers?

....

....

What emotion did I chose as my driver when I came home today?

....

....

What emotion did I choose to end my day?

....

....

Date ....

Random thoughts about your bus today:

....

....

....

....

....

....

....

....

....

....

....

....

....

....

....

....

....

....

....

....

Date ....

What emotion/s were driving when you woke up today?

....

....

What emotion/s did I choose to be my driver for my morning?

....

....

Did my emotions get triggered today and hijack my bus? If so, what was the trigger?

....

....

What drivers did I chose throughout my day? Were they my most resourceful drivers?

....

....

What emotion did I chose as my driver when I came home today?

....

....

What emotion did I choose to end my day?

....

....

Date ....

Random thoughts about your bus today:

....

....

....

....

....

....

....

....

....

....

....

....

....

....

....

....

....

....

Date ....

What emotion/s were driving when you woke up today?

....

....

What emotion/s did I choose to be my driver for my
morning?

....

....

Did my emotions get triggered today and hijack my
bus? If so, what was the trigger?

....

....

What drivers did I chose throughout my day? Were
they my most resourceful drivers?

....

....

What emotion did I chose as my driver when I came
home today?

....

....

What emotion did I choose to end my day?

....

....

Date ....

Random thoughts about your bus today:

....

....

....

....

....

....

....

....

....

....

....

....

....

....

....

....

....

....

....

Date ....

What emotion/s were driving when you woke up today?

....

....

What emotion/s did I choose to be my driver for my morning?

....

....

Did my emotions get triggered today and hijack my bus? If so, what was the trigger?

....

....

What drivers did I chose throughout my day? Were they my most resourceful drivers?

....

....

What emotion did I chose as my driver when I came home today?

....

....

What emotion did I choose to end my day?

....

....

Date ....

Random thoughts about your bus today:

....

....

....

....

....

....

....

....

....

....

....

....

....

....

....

....

....

....

....

Date ....

What emotion/s were driving when you woke up today?

....

....

What emotion/s did I choose to be my driver for my morning?

....

....

Did my emotions get triggered today and hijack my bus? If so, what was the trigger?

....

....

What drivers did I chose throughout my day? Were they my most resourceful drivers?

....

....

What emotion did I chose as my driver when I came home today?

....

....

What emotion did I choose to end my day?

....

....

Date ....

Random thoughts about your bus today:

....

....

....

....

....

....

....

....

....

....

....

....

....

....

....

....

....

....

....

....

Date ....

What emotion/s were driving when you woke up today?

....

....

What emotion/s did I choose to be my driver for my morning?

....

....

Did my emotions get triggered today and hijack my bus? If so, what was the trigger?

....

....

What drivers did I chose throughout my day? Were they my most resourceful drivers?

....

....

What emotion did I chose as my driver when I came home today?

....

....

What emotion did I choose to end my day?

....

....

Date ....

Random thoughts about your bus today:

....

....

....

....

....

....

....

....

....

....

....

....

....

....

....

....

....

....

....

Date ....

What emotion/s were driving when you woke up today?

....

....

What emotion/s did I choose to be my driver for my morning?

....

....

Did my emotions get triggered today and hijack my bus? If so, what was the trigger?

....

....

What drivers did I chose throughout my day? Were they my most resourceful drivers?

....

....

What emotion did I chose as my driver when I came home today?

....

....

What emotion did I choose to end my day?

....

....

Date ....

Random thoughts about your bus today:

....

....

....

....

....

....

....

....

....

....

....

....

....

....

....

....

....

....

....

Date ....

What emotion/s were driving when you woke up today?

....

....

What emotion/s did I choose to be my driver for my
morning?

....

....

Did my emotions get triggered today and hijack my
bus? If so, what was the trigger?

....

....

What drivers did I chose throughout my day? Were
they my most resourceful drivers?

....

....

What emotion did I chose as my driver when I came
home today?

....

....

What emotion did I choose to end my day?

....

....

Date ....

Random thoughts about your bus today:

....

....

....

....

....

....

....

....

....

....

....

....

....

....

....

....

....

....

....

Date ....

What emotion/s were driving when you woke up today?

....
....

What emotion/s did I choose to be my driver for my morning?

....
....

Did my emotions get triggered today and hijack my bus? If so, what was the trigger?

....
....

What drivers did I chose throughout my day? Were they my most resourceful drivers?

....
....

What emotion did I chose as my driver when I came home today?

....
....

What emotion did I choose to end my day?

....
....

Date ....

Random thoughts about your bus today:

....

....

....

....

....

....

....

....

....

....

....

....

....

....

....

....

....

....

....

Date ....

What emotion/s were driving when you woke up today?

....

....

What emotion/s did I choose to be my driver for my
morning?

....

....

Did my emotions get triggered today and hijack my
bus? If so, what was the trigger?

....

....

What drivers did I chose throughout my day? Were
they my most resourceful drivers?

....

....

What emotion did I chose as my driver when I came
home today?

....

....

What emotion did I choose to end my day?

....

....

Date ....

Random thoughts about your bus today:

....

....

....

....

....

....

....

....

....

....

....

....

....

....

....

....

....

....

....

....

Date ....

What emotion/s were driving when you woke up today?

....

....

What emotion/s did I choose to be my driver for my morning?

....

....

Did my emotions get triggered today and hijack my bus? If so, what was the trigger?

....

....

What drivers did I chose throughout my day? Were they my most resourceful drivers?   .

....

....

What emotion did I chose as my driver when I came home today?

....

....

What emotion did I choose to end my day?

....

....

Date ....

Random thoughts about your bus today:

....
....
....
....
....
....
....
....
....
....
....
....
....
....
....
....
....
....
....
....

Date ....

What emotion/s were driving when you woke up today?

....

....

What emotion/s did I choose to be my driver for my morning?

....

....

Did my emotions get triggered today and hijack my bus? If so, what was the trigger?

....

....

What drivers did I chose throughout my day? Were they my most resourceful drivers?

....

....

What emotion did I chose as my driver when I came home today?

....

....

What emotion did I choose to end my day?

....

....

Date ....

Random thoughts about your bus today:

....

....

....

....

....

....

....

....

....

....

....

....

....

....

....

....

....

....

....

....

Date ....

What emotion/s were driving when you woke up today?

....

....

What emotion/s did I choose to be my driver for my morning?

....

....

Did my emotions get triggered today and hijack my bus? If so, what was the trigger?

....

....

What drivers did I chose throughout my day? Were they my most resourceful drivers?

....

....

What emotion did I chose as my driver when I came home today?

....

....

What emotion did I choose to end my day?

....

....

Date ....

Random thoughts about your bus today:

....
....
....
....
....
....
....
....
....
....
....
....
....
....
....
....
....
....
....

Date ....

What emotion/s were driving when you woke up today?

....

....

What emotion/s did I choose to be my driver for my
morning?

....

....

Did my emotions get triggered today and hijack my
bus? If so, what was the trigger?

....

....

What drivers did I chose throughout my day? Were
they my most resourceful drivers?

....

....

What emotion did I chose as my driver when I came
home today?

....

....

What emotion did I choose to end my day?

....

....

Date ....

Random thoughts about your bus today:

....

....

....

....

....

....

....

....

....

....

....

....

....

....

....

....

....

....

....

Date ....

What emotion/s were driving when you woke up today?

....

....

What emotion/s did I choose to be my driver for my morning?

....

....

Did my emotions get triggered today and hijack my bus? If so, what was the trigger?

....

....

What drivers did I chose throughout my day? Were they my most resourceful drivers?

....

....

What emotion did I chose as my driver when I came home today?

....

....

What emotion did I choose to end my day?

....

....

Date ....

Random thoughts about your bus today:

....

....

....

....

....

....

....

....

....

....

....

....

....

....

....

....

....

....

....

....

Date ....

What emotion/s were driving when you woke up today?

....

....

What emotion/s did I choose to be my driver for my morning?

....

....

Did my emotions get triggered today and hijack my bus? If so, what was the trigger?

....

....

What drivers did I chose throughout my day? Were they my most resourceful drivers?

....

....

What emotion did I chose as my driver when I came home today?

....

....

What emotion did I choose to end my day?

....

....

Date ....

Random thoughts about your bus today:

....

....

....

....

....

....

....

....

....

....

....

....

....

....

....

....

....

....

....

Date ....

What emotion/s were driving when you woke up today?

....

....

What emotion/s did I choose to be my driver for my morning?

....

....

Did my emotions get triggered today and hijack my bus? If so, what was the trigger?

....

....

What drivers did I chose throughout my day? Were they my most resourceful drivers?

....

....

What emotion did I chose as my driver when I came home today?

....

....

What emotion did I choose to end my day?

....

....

Date ....

Random thoughts about your bus today:

....

....

....

....

....

....

....

....

....

....

....

....

....

....

....

....

....

....

....

....

Date ....

What emotion/s were driving when you woke up today?

....

....

What emotion/s did I choose to be my driver for my morning?

....

....

Did my emotions get triggered today and hijack my bus? If so, what was the trigger?

....

....

What drivers did I chose throughout my day? Were they my most resourceful drivers?

....

....

What emotion did I chose as my driver when I came home today?

....

....

What emotion did I choose to end my day?

....

....

Date ....

Random thoughts about your bus today:

....

....

....

....

....

....

....

....

....

....

....

....

....

....

....

....

....

....

....

Date ....

What emotion/s were driving when you woke up today?

....

....

What emotion/s did I choose to be my driver for my morning?

....

....

Did my emotions get triggered today and hijack my bus? If so, what was the trigger?

....

....

What drivers did I chose throughout my day? Were they my most resourceful drivers?

....

....

What emotion did I chose as my driver when I came home today?

....

....

What emotion did I choose to end my day?

....

....

Date ....

Random thoughts about your bus today:

....

....

....

....

....

....

....

....

....

....

....

....

....

....

....

....

....

....

....

Date ....

What emotion/s were driving when you woke up today?

....

....

What emotion/s did I choose to be my driver for my morning?

....

....

Did my emotions get triggered today and hijack my bus? If so, what was the trigger?

....

....

What drivers did I chose throughout my day? Were they my most resourceful drivers?

....

....

What emotion did I chose as my driver when I came home today?

....

....

What emotion did I choose to end my day?

....

....

Date ....

Random thoughts about your bus today:

....

....

....

....

....

....

....

....

....

....

....

....

....

....

....

....

....

....

....

Date ....

What emotion/s were driving when you woke up today?

....

....

What emotion/s did I choose to be my driver for my morning?

....

....

Did my emotions get triggered today and hijack my bus? If so, what was the trigger?

....

....

What drivers did I chose throughout my day? Were they my most resourceful drivers?

....

....

What emotion did I chose as my driver when I came home today?

....

....

What emotion did I choose to end my day?

....

....

Date ....

Random thoughts about your bus today:

....

....

....

....

....

....

....

....

....

....

....

....

....

....

....

....

....

....

....

....

Date ....

What emotion/s were driving when you woke up today?

....

....

What emotion/s did I choose to be my driver for my morning?

....

....

Did my emotions get triggered today and hijack my bus? If so, what was the trigger?

....

....

What drivers did I chose throughout my day? Were they my most resourceful drivers?

....

....

What emotion did I chose as my driver when I came home today?

....

....

What emotion did I choose to end my day?

....

....

Date ....

Random thoughts about your bus today:

....

....

....

....

....

....

....

....

....

....

....

....

....

....

....

....

....

....

....

Date ....

What emotion/s were driving when you woke up today?

....

....

What emotion/s did I choose to be my driver for my morning?

....

....

Did my emotions get triggered today and hijack my bus? If so, what was the trigger?

....

....

What drivers did I chose throughout my day? Were they my most resourceful drivers?

....

....

What emotion did I chose as my driver when I came home today?

....

....

What emotion did I choose to end my day?

....

....

Date ....

Random thoughts about your bus today:

....

....

....

....

....

....

....

....

....

....

....

....

....

....

....

....

....

....

....

Date ....

What emotion/s were driving when you woke up today?

....

....

What emotion/s did I choose to be my driver for my morning?

....

....

Did my emotions get triggered today and hijack my bus? If so, what was the trigger?

....

....

What drivers did I chose throughout my day? Were they my most resourceful drivers?

....

....

What emotion did I chose as my driver when I came home today?

....

....

What emotion did I choose to end my day?

....

....

Date ....

Random thoughts about your bus today:

....

....

....

....

....

....

....

....

....

....

....

....

....

....

....

....

....

....

....

Date ....

What emotion/s were driving when you woke up today?

....

....

What emotion/s did I choose to be my driver for my morning?

....

....

Did my emotions get triggered today and hijack my bus? If so, what was the trigger?

....

....

What drivers did I chose throughout my day? Were they my most resourceful drivers?

....

....

What emotion did I chose as my driver when I came home today?

....

....

What emotion did I choose to end my day?

....

....

Date ....

Random thoughts about your bus today:

....

....

....

....

....

....

....

....

....

....

....

....

....

....

....

....

....

....

....

Date ....

What emotion/s were driving when you woke up today?

....

....

What emotion/s did I choose to be my driver for my morning?

....

....

Did my emotions get triggered today and hijack my bus? If so, what was the trigger?

....

....

What drivers did I chose throughout my day? Were they my most resourceful drivers?

....

....

What emotion did I chose as my driver when I came home today?

....

....

What emotion did I choose to end my day?

....

....

Date ....

Random thoughts about your bus today:

....

....

....

....

....

....

....

....

....

....

....

....

....

....

....

....

....

....

....

....

Date ....

What emotion/s were driving when you woke up today?

....

....

What emotion/s did I choose to be my driver for my morning?

....

....

Did my emotions get triggered today and hijack my bus? If so, what was the trigger?

....

....

What drivers did I chose throughout my day? Were they my most resourceful drivers?

....

....

What emotion did I chose as my driver when I came home today?

....

....

What emotion did I choose to end my day?

....

....

Date ....

Random thoughts about your bus today:

....

....

....

....

....

....

....

....

....

....

....

....

....

....

....

....

....

....

....

Date ....

What emotion/s were driving when you woke up today?

....

....

What emotion/s did I choose to be my driver for my
morning?

....

....

Did my emotions get triggered today and hijack my
bus? If so, what was the trigger?

....

....

What drivers did I chose throughout my day? Were
they my most resourceful drivers?

....

....

What emotion did I chose as my driver when I came
home today?

....

....

What emotion did I choose to end my day?

....

....

Date ....

Random thoughts about your bus today:

....

....

....

....

....

....

....

....

....

....

....

....

....

....

....

....

....

What have you learned about yourself on this
journey?

Absorbed
Abhorrence
Acceptance
Admiration
Adoration
Adrift
Aching
Affection
Afraid
Agitated
Agony
Aggravated
Alarm
Alert
Alienated
Alive
Alone
Amazed
Amused
Anger
Angst
Animated
Animosity
Animus
Annoyed
Antagonistic
Anticipation
Antipathy
Antsy
Anxiety
Apathetic
Apologetic
Appalled
Appreciative
Apprehensive
Ardor
Arousal
Astonishment
Astounded
Attachment
Attraction
Aversion
Awe
Awkward
Baffled

Bashful
Befuddled
Bemused
Betrayed
Bewildered
Bitter
Blessed
Bliss
Blithe
Blue
Bold
Bonhomie
Boredom
Bothered
Bouncy
Brave
Breathless
Brooding
Bubbly
Buoyant
Burning
Calm
Captivated
Carefree
Caring
Cautious
Certain
Chagrin
Challenged
Chary
Cheerful
Choked
Choleric
Clueless
Cocky
Cold
Collected
Comfortable
Commiseration
Committed
Compassionate
Complacent
Complaisance
Composed
Compunction

Confused
Courage
Concerned
Confident
Conflicted
Consternation
Contemplative
Contempt
Contentment
Contrition
Cordial
Cowardly
Crafty
Cranky
Craving
Crestfallen
Cross
Cruel
Crummy
Crushed
Curious
Cynical
Defeated
Dejection
Delectation
Delighted
Delirious
Denial
Derisive
Desire
Desolation
Despair
Despondent
Detached
Determined
Detestation
Devastated
Devotion
Disappointed
Disbelief
Disdain
Disgruntled
Disgust
Disillusioned
Disinterested

Dismay
Distaste
Distracted
Distress
Disturbed
Doleful
Dopey
Doubtful
Down
Downcast
Drained
Dread
Dubious
Dumbfounded
Eager
Earnest
Ease
Ebullient
Ecstatic
Edgy
Elated
Embarrassment
Empathic
Empty
Enchantment
Energetic
Engrossed
Enjoyment
Enlightenment
Enmity
Entertainment
Enthralled
Enthusiasm
Envy
Euphoria
Exasperated
Excitement
Excluded
Exhausted
Exhilaration
Expectant
Exuberant
Fanatical
Fascinated
Fatigued

Feisty
Felicitous
Fervor
Flabbergasted
Floored
Fondness
Foolish
Foreboding
Fortunate
Frazzled
Free
Fretful
Frightened
Frustrated
Fulfilled
Furious
Genial
Giddy
Glad
Gleeful
Gloomy
Goofy
Gratified
Grateful
Greedy
Grief
Groggy
Grudging
Guarded
Guilt
Gung-ho
Gusto
Hankering
Happy
Harassed
Hatred
Heartache
Heartbroken
Helpless
Hesitant
Hollow
Homesick
Hopeful
Horrified
Hostile

Humiliated
Humored
Hurt
Hyper
Hysterical
Impatient
Incensed
Indifferent
Indignant
Infatuated
Inferior
Inspired
Intense
Interested
Intimacy
Intimidated
Intoxicated
Intrigued
Introspective
Invigorated
Irascible
Ire
Irritated
Isolated
Jaded
Jealous
Jittery
Jocular
Jocund
Jolly
Jovial
Joy
Jubilant
Jumpy
Keen
Lazy
Left out
Lethargic
Liberation
Lighthearted
Liking
Listless
Lively
Lonely
Longing

Lost
Love
Lucky
Lust
Mad
Meditative
Melancholic
Mellow
Merry
Miffed
Mirth
Mischievous
Miserable
Mollified
Mortified
Motivated
Mournful
Moved
Mystified
Nasty
Nauseous
Needy
Nervous
Neutral
Nonplussed
Nostalgic
Numb
Obsessed
Offended
Optimistic
Outrage
Overwhelmed
Pacified
Pain
Panic
Paranoid
Passion
Pathetic
Peaceful
Peevish
Pensive
Perky
Perplexed
Perturbed
Pessimistic

Petrified
Petty
Petulant
Phlegmatic
Pity
Playful
Pleasure
Positive
Possessive
Powerful
Powerless
Preoccupied
Protective
Proud
Psyched
Pumped
Puzzled
Quizzical
Rage
Rapture
Rattled
Reassured
Receptive
Reflective
Regret
Relaxed
Relief
Relish
Reluctance
Remorse
Repugnance
Resentment
Resignation
Restless
Revolted
Sad
Sanguine
Satisfied
Scandalized
Scorn
Secure
Self-Conscious
Selfish
Sensual
Sensitive

Serendipitous
Serene
Settled
Shaken
Shame
Sheepish
Shock
Shy
Sick
Silly
Sincere
Skeptical
Sluggish
Smug
Snappy
Solemn
Solicitous
Somber
Sore
Sorrow
Sorry
Sour
Speechless
Spiteful
Sprightly
Stirred
Stressed
Strong
Stung
Stunned
Stupefied
Submissive
Succor
Suffering
Suffocated
Sullen
Sunny
Superior
Sure
Surprised
Startled
Sympathy
Tenderness
Tense
Terror

Testy
Tetchy
Thankful
Thirst
Thoughtful
Thrill
Timid
Tired
Vexation
Vigilant
Vindication
Vindictive
Warmth
Wary
Weak
Weary
Welcome
Woe
Wonder
Woozy
Worry
Wrath
Wretched
Yearning
Zeal
Zest

Titillation
Tormented
Torn
Torture
Touched
Traumatized
Tranquil
Trepidation

Triumphant
Troubled
Trust
Twitchy
Upbeat
Upset
Uptight
Vehement

"The best and most beautiful things in the world cannot be seen or even touched. They must be felt with the heart" - *Helen Keller*

Made in the USA
Middletown, DE
05 February 2020

84168660R00073